What the Wind Showed to Me

By Emma Rose Sparrow

Editor-in-Chief: Connor Chagnon
Sterling Elle Publishing
Bradford, Massachusetts
ISBN: 1500664685
ISBN-13: 978-1500664688

WHAT THE WIND SHOWED TO ME

An Emma Rose Sparrow Book

WHAT THE WIND SHOWED TO ME follows the story of a woman who expects to have a ho-hum day. But she finds that if you just take a closer look, surprises and beauty can be seen everywhere.

It all begins when a breeze picks up a feather and brings her along on an enlightening journey.

If you are an adult bookworm who is looking for an interesting read or a book lover that enjoys a book that can be read over and over, this book is for you.

It is hoped that you find this book worthy of adding to your collection.

Enjoy your read!

OTHER BOOKS IN THIS SERIES BY EMMA ROSE SPARROW

A Dusting of Snow

The Sandy Shoreline

*Look for more titles coming soon!

TABLE OF CONTENTS

ACKNOWLEDGMENTS

Books allow a person to travel, while they stay sitting comfortably in place. I have journeyed to many locations in my lifetime, all from the coziness of my favorite sofa or my bed. I am sure you have too.

For this reason I wish to thank all of the authors in the world for giving us great book collections to choose from.

Also, a huge "thank you" is sent out to all of the amazing bookworms around the globe. It is your love of reading that inspires authors to write.

If you are a book lover, thank you for your interest in reading. I'm sure that you'll agree that books are one of the best forms of entertainment.

~ Emma Rose Sparrow

CHAPTER 1: THE FEATHER

When I woke up, the first thing that I thought about was how I wanted breakfast. I could smell eggs and bacon cooking. Maybe it was just my imagination, since I woke up so hungry. Or maybe someone was already starting to prepare the first meal of the day. Either way, eggs and bacon were in my near future and that made me happy.

The second thing that I thought about was the weather. Would it be raining? Rainy days can be wonderful if you feel like staying indoors and watch nature do its work. I know that it's beneficial for the trees and flowers to receive a good soaking every now and then. I didn't hear the pitter-patter of rain on the roof, so I assumed that any rainfall was at least holding off for now.

Would I see the first snowfall of the

season? Snow could be expected any day now. Maybe there would be a light dusting. Snow can look so beautiful, but I wasn't ready for winter yet. I was looking for something else. I was hoping for a cool, sunny day.

I dressed and brushed my teeth. After a satisfying breakfast of bacon and eggs, I was ready to see what Mother Nature had in store for me. You just never know with her! Instead of peeking out of a window, I decided to face it head on.

When I stepped outside, I immediately smiled. There would be sunshine today. A few white puffy clouds slowly edged their way across the sky. The early morning sunlight appeared welcoming.

The late autumn air felt crisp and clean. It was just cool enough, that taking in a deep breath felt cleansing. It was the type of seasonal day that made you think about apple trees. And warm apple cider.

It was also very windy. And that is just the sort of day I truly enjoy. I closed my eyes for a moment. A strong breeze tousled my hair a bit; the air felt fresh against my face. There was a rustling of air rushing through the trees.

Oh, how I enjoyed hearing the cool breezes whip over the branches and leaves. It is a unique sound and I find it to be soothing. I stayed like that, eyes closed and focused on the whispering noises of the wind for a while.

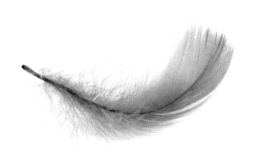

When I opened my eyes, something caught my attention. At first, I saw it from the corner of my eye and couldn't quite make it out. But something was floating in the air.

I stood in place and studied it further. Oh! It was a feather. A beautiful pearl white and gray feather.

The breeze captured the feather just perfectly. It twirled and spun in the air like a tiny helicopter that hovered in circles.

Wanting a closer look, I slipped on my shoes and jacket as I prepared to venture out further. Carefully walking over to the hovering feather, I hoped that the wind would not sweep it too high in the sky. This feather had piqued my interest.

CHAPTER 2: THE PERFECT PINK

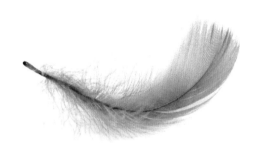

I stood in amazement at how the wind gracefully kept this feather in the air right above my head. I didn't try to reach up and grab it. My plan was to allow the wind to do as it wished.

Just as I wondered if this feather would forever linger in the same place, the breezed slowly moved it along. I followed.

Lifting and dipping, it remained airborne, gently gliding above the grass. My eyes followed its route as I made my way along to trail beneath it. It drifted over to a grouping of bushes. I smiled, as I happily walked over to see where this feather decided to take a rest.

It had settled itself down upon an array of bright green shrubbery. I leaned over to have a closer look. It seemed as if the feather was pointing and saying, "Here, take a look!"

I should tell you that I believe that all flowers are beautiful. But the one that this feather settled near was spectacular in every sense of the word.

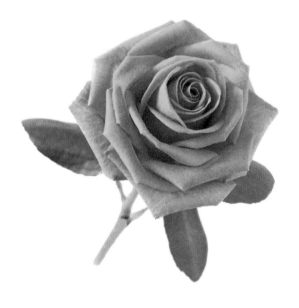

It was the most vibrant pink that nature could create. It had a swirl of impeccable petals. Each fold of the flower looked dewy soft. It was shiny and wonderfully silky. If I had to choose a name to describe this pink, I would have called it "perfect pink".

Researchers have found that the sight of flowers can elevate a person's mood. Just seeing a flower is said to increase happiness levels. I do believe it was working! I definitely felt cheerful.

Smelling a flower is said to make a person feel calm and relaxed. I wanted to test that theory.

Very carefully, I dipped my nose down to the pink bloom. I breathed in its scent. It was light, soft and refreshing.

Its aroma was like a delicate perfume. Not too overpowering but certainly a treat to my nose!

I thought for a moment about how flowers are the universal gift to all of us. They always comfort the receiver. Flowers are nature's way of making a person smile and feel loved.

The wind picked up a bit. As the feather wiggled in the breeze, I said a silent "thank you" to it. Beautiful flowers like this pink rose are present in nature all over the world. And these flowers belong to all of us. For that I was grateful.

As if tempting me to follow along, the feather wobbled again and the wind sent it soaring off once more. Where would the breeze bring it this time?

CHAPTER 3: A FLUTTERING

I was in a great mood, having seen the exceptional pink rose. But I was curious as to what I might spy next if I followed the feather. It was still darting and dipping in the breeze.

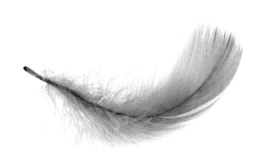

My eyes trailed its movements as I slowly walked in its direction.

Could it be going over to the lower branches of a small Birch tree? Yes! I was right. I stood patiently, watching this feather gently glide downward. It finished its journey by resting on a flaky, silvery branch.

I adjusted my eyeglasses as I took a step

closer. Ferns and frond created a shaded area for these low branches. A flutter of movement caused me to raise my eyebrows in surprise.

Somehow, this lovely little feather had floated over to show me another treat. There was the most remarkable butterfly; now sitting motionless on the curved branch.

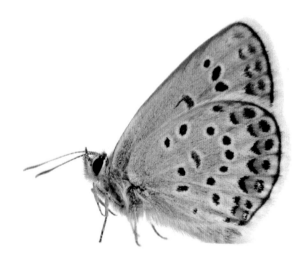

I had read somewhere that there are over 12,000 types of butterflies all over the world. I also read that there are perhaps thousands of more butterfly species that have not yet been identified. But I knew what this dazzling little creature was.

This butterfly was a Silver-studded Blue. The classy name of it is Plebejus argus. Sometimes people refer to it as a Hairstreak Butterfly.

It stood proudly, as if it were showing off the jazziest of outfits. Delicate and soft, it held its pose for me to study its beauty.

The outer edge of its exquisite wings were an amazing row of orange and black ovals. Small black spots dotted the center of the wings over a background of silky silver.

Most amazing was how the glossy silver graduated into a glistening pale blue.

I have seen a lot of butterflies in my lifetime. Usually I glance at them and think, "How pretty" and then go about my day.

This day was different. I stood for quite a while, in awe of how much beauty can exist. I thought about how lucky I was to be able to see this for myself.

The butterfly shook its bottom and fluttered off. I said a silent, "Thank you!" to it for allowing me to have an up close look at its loveliness.

As the butterfly flew off on its own journey, the feather lifted off as well. A gust of wind had swept in. Once again, this feather was leading me to the next stop.

CHAPTER 4: SEVEN DOTS

The wind that carried the feather swept it toward the ground. For a moment, I thought that maybe this little journey had ended. Like a popped balloon, it swayed downward onto the lawn. I supposed that I couldn't expect that this feather was to float around forever.

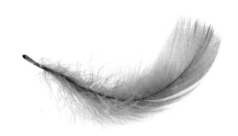

Maybe I should have gone back inside. But I didn't. I leaned over to have a closer look as the feather nestled itself in the soft, dewy grass.

I searched the area. For some reason, I had a strong feeling that if I looked close enough, there would be something to be seen!

Just as I began to think, "There's nothing

here", I spotted something tiny in the lush grass.

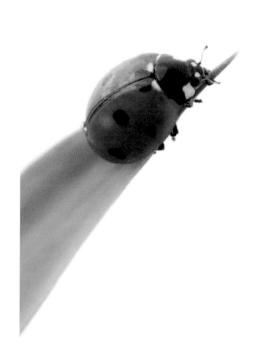

There, like a koala bear clung to a eucalyptus tree, was a ladybug clung to a single green blade.

There are over 5000 varieties of ladybugs all over the world. Some have as few as 2 dots. And some have as many as 15 dots. This little lady (or guy) had the classic red wings with 7 perfect black dots.

It was sturdy and fat but delicate at the same time. How delightful!

I have heard that some people call these the Lady Beetle or Ladybird Beetle. Personally, I always refer to these as Ladybugs.

Cultures all around the world consider this little insect to be a sign of good luck. Back in the Middle Ages, people wrote poems that praised Ladybugs for helping crops grow strong.

Hundreds of years ago, people would sing songs to Ladybugs. They believed doing so would bring a favorable harvest season to farms. The belief that Ladybugs bring good luck has stayed with us for generations.

I thought about trying to coax the Ladybug to crawl onto my finger. After all, I wanted to have good luck. But I decided that seeing it would be sufficient, since I didn't want to scare it away.

I marveled at the amazing beauty of this

little creature for a while. It was simply divine! Then, I looked down to the feather that had drifted in the breeze to bring me to the Ladybug.

The breeze caused the feather to struggle a bit in the blades of grass. Would the wind be strong enough to pick it up one more time? Or would it stay down in the lawn? As if it were being tugged by a string, it was airborne once again.

CHAPTER 5: BROWN SPIRALS

Carried by the breeze, the feather floated haphazardly through the air, as if it were trying to decide where to go next.

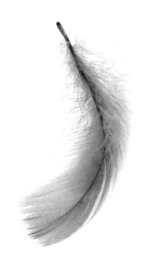

The wind was so erratic; I had no idea which direction it would send this wonderful, mysterious feather.

I was enjoying my journey and didn't want it to end quite yet.

With a pause and then a dip, it headed back toward my residence. With one more descending gust, it settled down onto a potted Hydrangea plant. I had noticed the other day that it was blooming quite well. The Hydrangea is really a very beautiful flower and one of my favorite.

This Hydrangea was a light lavender and rather full. But something was different today. There was a little visitor to this plant.

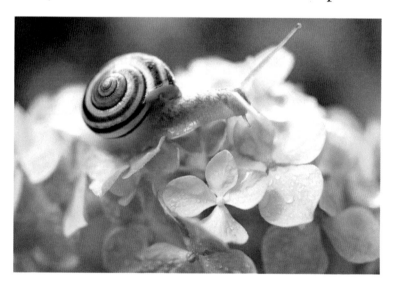

I was surprised to see a tiny garden snail. This snail is commonly known as a European Brown Garden Snail, even though it can be found in North America and other places outside of Europe. Its "fancy" name is Helix aspersa.

The garden snail is known for its small size and cream-colored shell with brown spiral stripes.

It's a bit mystifying how spirals can show up in so many diverse places. Here it was on this tiny snail. It is also the pattern of hurricanes when viewed from above. And galaxies are formed in a spiral shape. Nature is quite amazing, don't you agree?

Now, some people think that snails can be pests, since they eat away at plants. I thought about that for a moment. This tiny snail was not bothering anyone. Should I move him from the Hydrangea? It was a dilemma, for sure.

I decided to carefully pick him up and place him down onto a fallen leaf. That would keep the Hydrangea safe from his tiny mouth and he would be happy to munch away at the foliage.

I had almost forgotten about the feather that had floated through the air and brought me to this snail. Only when the wind whipped at my hair, did I remember.

Another gust of wind swept in and off the feather went again. I had spent a good amount of time on this journey so far. But I was not tired out yet. I felt as if I had a lot of energy. The cool air and refreshing breeze invigorated me. I didn't feel like going back in quite yet.

So, I decided that I would remain following the feather. What else was there to see today?

CHAPTER 6: MY CHUBBY LITTLE FRIEND

Carried by the wind, the feather drifted along as if it didn't have a care in the world. I didn't have to try to run after it; the feather was in no rush.

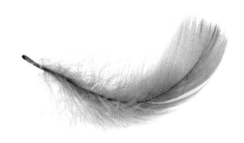

I didn't have to wait for it either; the feather made its way over the grass in a bumbling sort of manner.

I let out a soft laugh. It had just occurred to me that the feather reminded me of a clumsy tour guide.

It finally fluttered down upon a bench. I jokingly thought that maybe it wanted me to take a rest.   "Okay," I thought to myself, "I'll take a rest if you insist."   I sat myself down upon the faded warm wood of the bench.

I glanced around at my surroundings. There was peaceful ambiance.   I could hear birds chirping away in the distance.   An airplane was somewhere overhead; far away but close enough for me to hear the purr of its engines.   A few cars could be heard off in the distance, but not close enough to be a nuisance.

The sun sent out waves of warmth on this cool, autumn morning.   I took in a deep breath, savoring the peace and serenity of the day.   While some days could be hectic and some left me bored to tears, this day was utterly enjoyable.   Could it be any more perfect?

I received my answer as I heard a fluttering of wings.

A stunning bird gracefully landed on a branch, right across from where I sat!

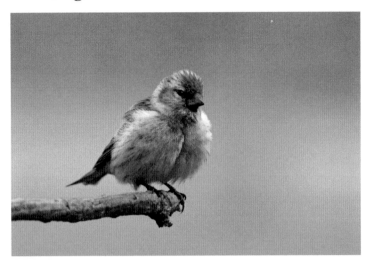

Oh, this little creature was chubby! It must have been young, as its feathers seemed quite soft and downy.

It was a Redpoll bird; an amazing songbird that travels in flocks of hundreds. But this little guy was sitting all alone.

These charming birds are known for their unique coloring. Both males and females have a bright red patch on the forehead. But this was a young male, as it also had a brilliant feathering of red on its chest.

It just sat there.   Staring at me.   I wished that I had a worm to offer this plump little guy.   I made a promise to myself to bring out some birdseed the next chance I had.

These birds are known to have an energetic "zapping" call.   And I soon found out why they call it that.   My feathered friend let out a delightful serious of soft, rapid calls.

It didn't sound like a "chirp".   It sounded more like a "Dreeee!".   Very distinctive indeed!

He looked right into my eyes, as if he wanted to say something.   Then, with a quick nod, he lifted up his wings and soared away into the treetops.   He was undoubtedly joining his friends in the safe haven of the forest.

CHAPTER 7: THE BEAUTY OF IT ALL

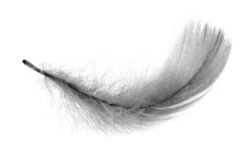

I remained on the bench, looking down at the feather that had started me on this little journey. It sat curled a bit, as if waiting to take off once again with the next gust of wind.

I thought about how there is so beauty all around us; we just need to stop and take a look. Had it not been for this feather, I wouldn't have stopped to take in the beauty of the rose, the butterfly, the Ladybug, the tiny snail or the bird.

As if right on cue, a huge gust of wind blew in and swept the feather up in its strength. It soared high into the sky. I watched it become smaller and smaller as it drifted out of view.

I might never see that feather again, and maybe it was on its way to offer a journey to someone else now. But I knew that from that day forward, I would take a bit of time to admire all that nature offers to us.

And I do hope I see that chubby little Redpoll bird again!

ABOUT THE AUTHOR

Emma Rose Sparrow lives in a small New England coastal town with her two sons. She enjoys many creative ventures, including design and writing. She wishes to personally thank each and every one of her book readers for keeping the art of reading alive.

OTHER BOOKS IN THIS SERIES BY EMMA ROSE SPARROW

A Dusting of Snow

The Sandy Shoreline

Look for more titles coming soon!

Made in the USA
Middletown, DE
05 November 2021

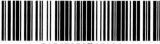